MW00618718

# High-Tech Pain Management for Pets

## Low-Level Laser Therapy
User's Manual for Veterinarians

Dr. Tamara S. Shearer

Edited by Stanford Apseloff

# High-Tech Pain Management for Pets

## Low-Level Laser Therapy
User's Manual for Veterinarians

Dr. Tamara S. Shearer

Edited by Stanford Apseloff

OHIO DISTINCTIVE PUBLISHING

Columbus, Ohio

Ohio Distinctive Publishing, Inc.
6500 Fiesta Drive, Columbus OH 43235
www.ohio-distinctive.com

© 2004 by Tamara S. Shearer and Stanford Apseloff
All rights reserved.  Published 2004.

Printed in the United States of America.

10 09 08 07 06 05 04    10 9 8 7 6 5 4 3 2 1

Photographs by Stanford Apseloff
Appendix Photographs by Dr. Tamara S. Shearer

ISBN:    0-9647934-5-8

Library of Congress Control Number:    2004101714

# ABOUT THE AUTHOR

Dr. Shearer owns and operates an innovative small-animal veterinary practice with a focus on applying new, noninvasive techniques to improve pet health care. In addition, she is a university guest lecturer and makes frequent appearances on local television as a veterinary advisor.

Dr. Shearer is the founder of the nonprofit Pet Hospice and Education Center, an organization dedicated to providing care and comfort to chronically and terminally ill pets. The Center also offers classes on pet first aid and pet geriatric care, and pet-care classes for children. In addition, Dr. Shearer has started a number of local neighborhood programs to promote animal welfare, including the Rusty Ranger Club (to educate children about pets) and a lost pet block-watch program. She is the veterinary advisor to a canine search-and-rescue group that participated in the 9/11 rescue efforts.

Dr. Shearer is the author of four other books: *Emergency First Aid For Your Dog*, *Emergency First Aid for Your Dog Handbook*, *Emergency First Aid for Your Cat*, and *The Essential Book for Dogs Over Five*.

Dr. Shearer is the recipient of the Hartz® "Veterinarian of the Year" award.

# PREFACE AND DISCLAIMER

As a practicing veterinarian, I have always been open to new concepts and new treatments regarding veterinary care. In my practice we use the best equipment available, including endoscopes, ultrasound equipment, and surgical lasers. In 2002, at a national veterinary conference, I was introduced to the low-level laser, and I have been using it ever since. In addition to the multitude of studies that extol the benefits of this high-tech treatment, I witness first-hand the results of its use in my practice on a daily basis. Although anecdotal evidence does not qualify as "proof", I know of no placebo effect in dogs and cats, and yet I most definitely see positive effects. For me, seeing is believing, and I am definitely a believer in low-level laser therapy. I use it in conjunction with other treatments, NOT in place of other treatments, to provide my patients with the best possible care I know how to give. Please note, however, that any claims that I make about the results of low-level laser therapy are based on my personal experience and my personal interpretation of the studies and research that I have investigated, and my statements throughout this book should be viewed as my opinions, beliefs and interpretations rather than established scientific facts. There are ample scientific studies (enough to satisfy the FDA) regarding certain specific benefits, but I leave it to you (and the FDA) to decide for yourselves what constitutes "proof" in any given treatment situation.

The content of this book is designed to be educational, but it is not designed to diagnose, treat or cure any disease. The content of this book consists of my opinions alone, and not those of the publisher, editor or any low-level laser manufacturer. My opinions are based on my experiences and my interpretations of those experiences, as well as my interpretations of research done by others.

The low-level lasers manufactured by 2035, Inc. that are discussed in this book have been registered with the FDA, but the FDA has not made a ruling as to their efficacy. The manufacturer of the low-level lasers discussed in this book did not take part in the writing of this book. The manufacturer makes no claims in this book, and no manufacturer claims should be inferred from this book.

# TABLE OF CONTENTS

# INTRODUCTION

In the past few years, great emphasis has been placed on making sure our pets are kept pain free. Veterinary studies confirm that pain can slow recoveries and even interfere with the immune systems of our pets. Recognizing the importance of pain management, progressive veterinary practices generally adopt a multimodal approach to increase the success of therapy to treat pain. Examples of this multimodal approach include combining drug therapy with supplements, proper diet, physical therapy, and/or acupuncture. Now there is another treatment to add to this multimodal approach to pain management, a remarkable high-tech treatment: the low-level laser.

A major advantage of low-level laser therapy is that it has no known side effects, and it complements other therapies. Its major benefits come in the form of improving recoveries by minimizing pain and expediting the healing process. Exciting information is being gathered about the ability of low-level lasers to work at a cellular level. Recently, the FDA approved low-level laser therapy devices to treat people with pain from carpal tunnel syndrome, neck pain and musculoskeletal pain. This recent approval has captured the attention of many professionals, including doctors, physical therapists, chiropractors, acupuncturists and veterinarians. Surprisingly, low-level lasers have been used successfully in Europe for more than thirty years.

The objective of this manual is to introduce veterinarians to low-level laser therapy, a technology that is offering new, high-tech treatment options for pets. This book will describe the history, safety, and applications of low-level laser in veterinary medicine. While this manual specifically describes use of four lasers by 2035, Inc., many techniques in this manual should be applicable to other low-level lasers as well. Consult your laser manufacturer regarding issues and questions that arise as you read this text.

# A BRIEF HISTORY AND DESCRIPTION OF LASERS

Einstein postulated a theory about light amplification in the early 1900's, but it was not until 1960 that Theodore Miaman developed the first ruby laser. Since then, many types of lasers have evolved that do a variety of jobs. Examples include surgical cutting lasers, industrial lasers, bar code readers, laser printers, laser engineering instruments, CD players, and the low-level laser for medical and veterinary use. The low-level laser has been used in Europe and Asia now for over thirty years.

The term "laser" stands for Light Amplification by Stimulated Emission of Radiation. Lasers work when an electrical current stimulates a specific element or medium to give off energy-rich photons. These energy-rich photons of a specific wavelength are then in a form that can be utilized for a variety of purposes.

Lasers that are used for veterinary purposes are applied to (i.e., have their beams placed directly over) specific areas of a pet's body. The pet's tissue reaction to a laser, ranging from mild stimulation to complete vaporization, is dependent upon six factors:

1. Laser class
2. Laser wavelength
3. Laser power
4. Laser beam (i.e., the relative focus or dispersion of the beam)
5. Exposure (i.e., duration of the laser beam)
6. Variability of the tissue exposed to the laser

The first three of these factors merit some additional discussion:

**LASER CLASS** – All lasers are classified by the FDA based on their safety to the eyes:

Class I. These lasers will do no harm to the eyes because they emit low optical radiation. Examples include laser printers and bar code readers. Some low-level lasers (e.g., the Q1000 and Q100 resonating lasers discussed on pages 15-16) are Class I lasers.

Class II. Momentary viewing of this class of lasers is not considered dangerous.

Class IIIa. With this class of lasers, direct viewing may be hazardous. Examples include laser pointers and some low-level lasers (e.g., the 660 Enhancer stimulating laser discussed on pages 15 and 17).

Class IIIb. Protective glasses must be worn to protect the eyes from accidental exposure. The 808 Enhancer low-level stimulating laser (discussed on pages 15 and 17) is a Class IIIb laser.

Class IV. These lasers can cause serious injury to eyes and skin. Surgical lasers are typically Class IV lasers.

Regardless of the laser's classification, make sure that a laser is never aimed into a person's or pet's eyes. At the time of this printing low-level laser studies show that because of their low energies, treatment of pets as directed with low-level lasers causes no known side effects.

**LASER WAVELENGTH** – The low-level lasers are made up of small semiconductor chips, like those in computers. The laser diodes are actually made in a vacuum by combining certain elements. Examples of the laser diodes discussed in this manual include: (1) indium, gallium, aluminum, and phosphrous (InGaAlP), which produce wavelengths from 630 to 685 nanometers (visible red light range), (2) gallium, aluminum, and arsenide (GaAlAs), which produce wavelengths ranging from 780 to 870 nanometers (near infrared), and (3) gallium and arsenide (GaAs), which produce wavelengths of 904 to 905 nanometers. A low-level laser operates on only one watt or less of power. By contrast, $CO_2$ cutting lasers commonly used for veterinary surgical procedures operate on 2-20 watts of power.

**LASER POWER** – There are two types of low-level lasers, and they are distinguished based on their power. Resonating lasers operate under 5 milliwatts of power, and they are primarily used for therapy on muscles, wounds and pain management. Examples include the Q1000 and Q100, both manufactured by 2035, Inc. Stimulating lasers operate from 5 milliwatts to 500 milliwatts of power. Examples of stimulating lasers include the 660 Enhancer and the 808 Enhancer, both manufactured by 2035, Inc. Compared to resonating lasers, stimulating lasers emit a more narrow beam of energy and deliver more energy in less time. Stimulating lasers are used in acupoint stimulation for pain management, and they can also be used on nerves, cartilage, muscle, tendons, and bone. They are also good for superficial scar reduction, and dental applications. Stimulating lasers are not programmed for use on organs and glands.

# GENERAL APPLICATION

The protocols in this manual are based on a vast number of research studies and on human protocols, as well as on clinical use at my practice and elsewhere. However, use of the low-level laser is, by its nature, an inexact science. Different veterinary patients respond differently, regardless of size, species, breed, or physical characteristics. For no apparent reason, a lower dose will work better on one patient, and a higher dose will work better on another. Therefore, it is important to note that all of the protocols for all of the conditions in this book will need to be adjusted on a case-by-case basis. Regardless of whether your patient is a cat or an elephant, you should start with the recommended protocol, but then adjust treatments up or down as you determine best, based on the results that you achieve.

You will note that the protocols detailed in the following pages often prescribe treatment with a combination of resonating and stimulating lasers. If you have only one type of laser, start by following the protocol for that laser. For those protocols where more than one mode is recommended, you may use one mode immediately after the other, or if you prefer, you may leave some gap in time between the use of different modes.

The protocols in this book are based on the use of lasers manufactured by 2035, Inc., which have multiple modes that have been preprogrammed at specific frequencies, or combinations of frequencies. If you are using a laser that requires you to program your frequencies, you will need to consult with the manufacturer to determine the frequencies that might work best for you. However, regardless of which low-level laser you use, the general principles remain the same: For any given condition, start with a base level of treatments recommended by this book or your laser manufacturer, and then make adjustments based on your individual patients and the results that you achieve.

# LASER CHOICES

Lasers discussed in this text are the Q1000 model, the Q100 model, the 660 Enhancer, and the 808 Enhancer, all manufactured by 2035, Inc. The Q100 model is essentially the same size and shape as the Q1000 and is used in a similar manner, but my experience with both is that the Q1000 is more versatile. (You will note that the photographs in this book that illustrate use of a resonating laser all show the Q1000 model in action rather than the Q100).

There are several low-level lasers currently available, but they do not all have the same technology and quality. The resonating laser you choose for treatment should have automatic regulation of power output to maintain consistency. Without this power regulating feature, when the batteries that power the unit lose their charge, there will be inconsistency that could affect the results of therapy. This book focuses on the 2035, Inc. lasers because these are the low-level lasers that I use in my practice. There are six reasons why I choose to use these particular low-level lasers:

1.  <u>Ease of Use</u> – Frequencies have been preprogrammed into a few modes, which means that the user simply selects one of these few modes rather than choosing from a broad range of frequencies and a near-infinite combination of frequencies. The learning curve is short.
2.  <u>Portablility</u> – They are lightweight and durable.
3.  <u>State-of-the-Art Technology</u> – They maintain the same frequency and power output regardless of whether the battery is fully charged. This feature is critical to ensuring consistency of treatment.
4.  <u>Affordable</u> – I found them to be less expensive than some other lasers that have fewer features.
5.  <u>Reproducible Effects</u> – My experience with these lasers is that they cause a predictable response to therapy.
6.  <u>Programmable Factory Options</u> – Although I have not taken advantage of this option, I know that the manufacturer can add an additional four modes to the Q1000 unit, and one additional mode to the Q100.

The following are the specifications for the 2035, Inc. low-level lasers at the time of this printing:

Specifications of the Q1000 (resonating laser)

| | |
|---|---|
| # of Lasers: | 12 |
| # LEDs: | 8 |
| Modes: | 3 preset, plus 4 optional |
| Frequency: | 1-160 Hertz |
| Wavelength: | multiple wavelengths from 470-940 nanometers |
| Power per Diode: | less than 5 milliwatts with a total maximum power of 42 milliwatts per 3-minute cycle |
| Total Output: | 3.9 Joules per 3-minute cycle |
| Power Density: | 2.4 milliwatts per square centimeter |
| Area: | 2.67 square inches |
| FDA Safety Class: | Class I |

The Q1000 has the capability of four additional modes that can be programmed at the factory. Each new mode can be programmed for up to eight frequencies.

These lasers are primarily used for therapy on muscles, wounds and pain management. The Q1000 is used to power the 660 Enhancer and 808 Enhancer.

Specifications of the Q100 (resonating laser)

| | |
|---|---|
| # of Lasers: | 4 |
| # LEDs: | 4 |
| Modes: | 2 preset, plus 1 optional |
| Frequency: | 7-60 Hertz |
| Wavelength: | multiple wavelengths from 650-940 nanometers |
| Power per Diode: | less than 5 milliwatts with a total maximum power of 14 milliwatts per 3-minute cycle |
| Total Output: | 1.3 Joules per 3-minute cycle |
| Power Density: | 2.4 milliwatts per square centimeter |
| Area: | 1.5 square inches |
| FDA Safety Class: | Class I |

The Q100 can be used in place of the Q1000 but cannot power the 660 and 808 Enhancers. The Q100 is not as powerful or as versatile as the Q1000. The Q100 has the capability of one additional mode that can be programmed at the factory. The new mode can be programmed for up to eight frequencies.

Specifications of the 660 Enhancer (stimulating laser)

| | |
|---|---|
| Wavelength: | 660 nanometers |
| Diode: | One 50 milliwatt red laser diode |
| Power: | 30 milliwatts |
| Total Output: | 6.6 Joules per 3-minute cycle |
| Area: | 3mm x 1cm |
| FDA Safety Class: | IIIa |

Recommended uses include acupoint stimulation, superficial scar therapy, and dental applications.

Stimulating lasers operate over 5 milliwatts to 500 milliwatts of power. The 660 Enhancer operates at 30 milliwatts. Compared to resonating lasers, stimulating lasers emit a much more narrow beam of energy and deliver more energy in less time. Stimulating lasers are not programmed for use on organs and glands (except indirectly through acupoint stimulation).

The Q1000 is used to power the 660 Enhancer.

Specifications of the 808 Enhancer (stimulating laser)

| | |
|---|---|
| Wavelength: | 808 nanometers |
| Diode: | One 500 milliwatt infrared laser diode |
| Power: | 300 milliwatts |
| Total Output: | 54 Joules per 3-minute cycle |
| Area: | 3mm x 1cm |
| FDA Safety Class: | IIIb |

Recommended uses include treatments for bones, cartilage, joints, tendons and nerves, and for dental applications and deep scar therapy.

As mentioned above, stimulating lasers operate in the range of 5 milliwatts to 500 milliwatts of power. The 808 Enhancer operates at 300 milliwatts. Stimulating lasers are not programmed for use on organs and glands (except indirectly through acupoint stimulation).

The Q1000 is used to power the 808 Enhancer.

Your choice of low-level lasers will not vary depending upon the type of patients you treat. Although the photographs in this book depict treatments for cats and dogs, these same lasers can be used to treat anything from rodents to race horses. Refer to Cellular Mechanisms of Action on pages 19 and 20 to understand better how the same laser can be used to treat a variety of different animals.

# CELLULAR MECHANISMS OF ACTION

Exciting information is being gathered about the ability of the low-level laser to work at a cellular level. Some of the research includes the following:

In the journal *Lasers in Medical Science*, a study of mouse muscle regeneration (Amaral et al. 2001) showed a greater concentration of mitochondria and increased muscle fiber area in muscles treated with a helium-neon laser at 2.6 Joules per square centimeter.

Another study (Karu et al. 2001) showed that the mechanism of low-level laser therapy at the cellular level is based on electronic excitation of chromophores in cytochrome c oxidase which modulates the redox status of molecules and enhances the functional activity.

Itoh, Murakami, Orihashi, and others (2000) showed that erythrocytes produced more adenosine triphosphate (ATP) and were more deformable after laser exposure. Their conclusion was that low-level laser treatment protected human erythrocytes from damage caused by artificial heart-lung machines.

Wilden and Karthein (1998) showed the influence of low-level laser irradiation on cellular energy transfer. They found increased ATP production in mitochondria stimulated by low-level laser light from the red and near infrared wavelengths.

In *Lasers in Surgery and Medicine*, Sroka, Schaffer, Fuchs, and others (1999) showed significantly increased mitotic rates of skeletal myotubes exposed to a laser with a wavelength of 635 nanometers.

In their study of human periodontal ligament fibroblasts, Kreisler, Christoffers, Willershausen, and d'Hoedt (2003) showed that cells irradiated with an 809-nanometer diode laser revealed a considerably higher proliferation activity than the control group.

In combination, a range of studies on use of the low-level laser suggests that low-level laser therapy may produce the following cellular mechanisms of action:

1. Increased cellular receptor activity
2. Influence on cell membrane permeability
3. Increased ATPase and activation of cAMP
4. Increased procollagen synthesis in fibroblasts
5. Activation of macrophages
6. Stimulation of the Na/K pump
7. Promotion of biostimulation of cells
8. Promotion of photostimulation of cells
9. Promotion of endogenous opiate production
10. Inhibition of bradykinin and leukotienes

# CLINICAL APPLICATIONS FOR PETS

Research studies show that low-level laser therapy may be applied in practice in a variety of ways. Currently there are more than 2000 publications on the study of low-level laser therapy. The majority of the studies shows a positive outcome.

In the publication *Clinical Rheumatology*, Ozdemir, Birtane, and Kokino (2001) performed a double-blind study in which people with cervical osteoarthritis (COA) responded positively to low-level laser treatments. They had significant improvement in the range of neck motion and function, and in the relief of pain, plus a decrease in paravertebral muscle spasms.

In a study at the Kyorin University School of Medicine in Japan, Kubota (2002) assessed the effects of low-level laser therapy on blood flow in skin flaps, which are used in reconstructive surgeries for tissue defects. He showed that blood flow and perfusion was enhanced in skin flaps exposed to an 830-nanometer diode laser. The same flaps also had significantly better survival rate compared to the control group.

In the journal *Lasers in Surgery and Medicine*, Rochkind, Nissan, Alon, and others (2001) showed that a low-level laser applied to the spinal cord may improve recovery of the corresponding peripheral nerve. The study involved crush injury to the sciatic nerve in rats. In the same issue of *Lasers in Surgery and Medicine*, Stadler, Lanzafame, Evans, and others (2001) showed an increase in wound tensile strength in diabetic mice when the wounds were treated with a laser operating at a wavelength of 830 nanometers.

At the University of Kansas, in the Department of Physical Therapy and Rehabilitation Sciences, research by Enwemeka and Reddy (2000-2001) showed that treatment using lasers with wavelengths of 632.8 and 904 nanometers may augment collagen synthesis, modulate the maturation of newly-synthesized collagen, and improve the biomechanical characterisitcs of repaired tendons.

Kreisler, Haj, Noroozi, and Willershausen (2004) showed in a study that people who had endodontic surgeries had reduced postoperative pain levels after treatment with an 809-nanometer laser at 50 milliwatts for 150 seconds right after suturing. Reduced pain levels, compared with the control group, were reported throughout the seven days after the surgery, and were most significant on the first postoperative day.

The studies on use of the low-level laser suggest that low-level laser therapy may produce some or all of the following results:

1. Speed bone repair
2. Reduce scarring
3. Reduce inflammation
4. Increase lymphatic drainage
5. Reduce pain
6. Improve healing time
7. Relax tight muscles
8. Increase mobility
9. Reduce swelling
10. Increase tendon and wound strength

# FACTS, GUIDELINES AND USE OF LOW-LEVEL LASERS

## FACTS

1. Low-level laser treatment will not mask physiologic indicators such as heart rate and respiratory rate nor hide deterioration from any disease process.
2. Resonating lasers (Q1000 and Q100) operate under 5 milliwatts of power. They are meant to be applied directly over the affected areas and are used for therapy on muscles and wounds, as well as for pain management.
3. Stimulating lasers (660 Enhancer and 808 Enhancer) operate from 5 milliwatts to 500 milliwatts of power. These lasers emit a narrow beam of energy and are used in acupuncture point stimulation for pain management. They may also be used on nerves, cartilage, muscle, tendons, and bone. They are also good for superficial scar reduction and dental applications.
4. Stimulating lasers are not programmed for use on organs and glands.

## GUIDELINES AND HELPFUL HINTS

1. Make your diagnosis prior to treatment.
2. Never look directly into a laser device. When using the laser on or near a pet's eyes, use a dry wash cloth to cover the pet's eyes to help prevent the pet from looking into the laser. (Note: the wash cloth will NOT shield the laser from the pet's eyes.)
3. Treat patients on a carpeted floor or otherwise padded surface.
4. When using the laser in an area prone to contamination (e.g., on an open wound), cover the laser with a disposible glove.
5. The area being treated does not need to be shaved. The laser will operate through hair and fur and even bandages.
6. It is not necessary to press the laser against the pet. When treating an extremely sensitive area (e.g., an open wound), place the laser within 1/2 inch of the area.
7. For musculoskeletal problems, make sure to treat on, above and below the painful area at the site of tendon and ligament origin and insertion.
8. If you are unsure of treatment timing, start with one treatment daily for three days, then one treatment every other day for three treatments, and then once weekly or every other week as

needed. Start with each treatment at three minutes duration regardless of the pet's size or condition, and make adjustments (plus or minus) based on your observed results.

9. If pain returns or healing slows, modify treatment time. Start with a modest increase in treatment time (e.g., 25%), and if that does not produce the desired effect, try reducing the treatment time instead (e.g., reduce 25% from the original treatment time).

10. Even if you are using a laser that maintains its output independent of battery power, make sure that you have enough battery power to do the job. Keep a spare charged battey available in case your primary battery runs out of power.

NOTE: If you are using a low-level laser manufactured by 2035, Inc., the unit will emit a consistent level of power regardless of the level of charge in the battery. It is not necessary to recharge the battery until the remaining charge is insufficient to power the unit. If you are using a low-level laser by another manufacturer, you should inquire about possible power fluctuation associated with battery charge.

Low-Level Laser Prescriptions for Pets

Resonating lasers (e.g., the Q1000 and Q100) are meant to be applied directly over the affected areas and are used for therapy on muscles and wounds, and for pain management. The Q1000 and the Q100 have preprogrammed frequencies in multiple modes (three modes for the Q1000 and two for the Q100). The Q1000 has mode frequencies preprogrammed for specific purposes:

Q1000 Mode 1. Use Mode 1 to decrease healing time of wounds, reduce pain and inflammation, and provide muscle relaxation.
Q1000 Mode 2. Use Mode 2 for reenergizing cells.
Q1000 Mode 3. Use Mode 3 for wounds, pain and inflammation, and to provide muscle relaxation. Studies show that the 29 frequencies in this mode may potentially have benefits with internal disease.

The Q100 has two modes only, and most of the protocols in this book use Mode 1 only.

The 660 Enhancer stimulating laser should be used on acupuncture and acupressure points. It can also be used for surface scars and dental procedures. The 808 Enhancer should be used over areas of joint/tendon pain and for bone/cartilage regeneration and deep scar reduction. Stimulating lasers (e.g., the 660 Enhancer and the 808 Enhancer) are not programmed for use on organs and glands.

# CONDITIONS

The low-level laser can, and should, be part of a multimodal approach to veterinary medicine. Use the low-level laser in addition to, NOT instead of, other treatments and therapies.

For your convenience, the following format is used for low-level laser protocols for each condition:

Q1000 or Q100 Laser Placement
Q1000 Mode and Time
Q100 Mode and Time
Use of 660 Enhancer
Use of 808 Enhancer
Frequency of Use

NOTE: In all instances, the protocols call for use of EITHER the Q1000 or the Q100, but not both. The Q1000 is preferable in all situations. Also, note that any protocol that specifies use of the 660 Enhancer and the 808 Enhancer is indicating that these Enhancers should be used in addition to the Q1000 or Q100. When both the 660 and the 808 Enhancers are listed in a protocol, both should be used (unless the protocol specifically indicates to use only one). If you have only one of the Enhancers, use what you have and ignore the protocol for the other. If you have no Enhancers, then use only the Q1000 or Q100 as specified.

There are many conditions detailed below that specify use of multiple lasers (e.g., the Q1000 plus the 660 Enhancer plus the 808 Enhancer). If you do not have access to all of the lasers, use what you have. My experience is that the effects of multiple low-level lasers seems to be cumulative, but longer is not necessarily better when it comes to use of each individual low-level laser. For any given situation, start with the "Base Time" specified in the protocol, and then, if you do not achieve the desired results, make minor adjustments within the specified time range. These minor adjustments should not be to either extreme end of the time range, but rather they should be plus or minus 25% to 50% of the Base Time. Your first adjustment, if any is necessary, should probably be to increase the time of treatment; if that yields no positive results, then try decreasing the treatment time.

Based on the response of each individual patient, and your experience in general, you might end up making a series of time adjustments in certain situations.

If the condition calls for use of the 660 Enhancer and/or 808 Enhancer in addition to the Q1000 or Q100, start with the Q1000 or Q100 and then immediately follow with the 660 and/or 808. For any given condition, apply the same "Frequency of Use" guidelines to the 660 and 808 (whenever their use is called for) as you do for the Q1000 or Q100. Also note that frequently the protocols call for use of two modes for the Q1000 (e.g., Mode 1 and Mode 3). In those situations, use the Q1000 on Mode 1 for the entire specified time, and then immediately switch to the second mode and repeat the procedure for the same specified time. (In other words, use the complete time for each mode.)

When acupuncture, acupressure and trigger points are being targeted for treatment by the 660 Enhancer, note that the Base Times specified in the protocols are for each such point. Also, note that Base Times are meant to apply to individual treatment sites, and multiple sites will therefore require multiple treatments for the specified Base Time. Also, if the area being treated is larger than the laser's treatment surface, then use the laser as many times as necessary to cover the entire treatment site. For example, if you are using the Q1000 to treat an abrasion that is a few inches long, you may need to use the Q1000 a few times to completely cover the abrasion. Note, however, that regarding the 660 Enhancer and the 808 Enhancer, in those instances where the protocol calls for use directly over a site, you should limit use of these devices to no more than two or three times the number of treatments from the Q1000 (or Q100). In other words, if you are treating a large abrasion with one of the Enhancers, and the abrasion requires two separate treatments with the Q1000 to cover the entire area of the abrasion, then limit your use of the Enhancer to no more than four or six treatments for that abrasion. While I recommend that you hold the Q1000 steady when treating any given area, I recommend that for use of the Enhancers on sites that are large, you should move the Enhancer a little every several seconds to treat an area of approximately 1/2 to 1 square inch per Base Time.

There may be conditions that you encounter that are not specifically addressed by this book. If that happens, use your best judgment based on your knowledge of the condition and your experience with the laser. Remember, at the time of this printing, there are no known adverse reactions or side effects from use of the low-level laser on pets. Therefore, if you have reason to believe that low-level laser treatment might be of benefit, there is every reason to err on the side of use.

The following pages provide treatment protocols for a variety of conditions. For your convenience, these conditions are listed in alphabetical order.

## ABRASIONS
Q1000 or Q100 Laser Placement:
Place directly over the abrasion and any surrounding soft tissues that may be experiencing pain from the lesion.

Q1000:  Mode 1
Base Time:  1 minute each site. (Range:  1/4 to 3 minutes)
or:
Q100:  Mode 1
Base Time:  3 minutes each site. (Range:  3/4 to 9 minutes)

In addition, use the 660 Enhancer for acupuncture or acupressure points and directly over and around a superficial abrasion.
Base Time: 1 minute. (Range:  1/2 to 2 minutes)

Use the 808 Enhancer directly over and around lesion if the abrasion is deep.
Base Time: 1 minute. (Range:  1/2 to 2 minutes)

Frequency of Use:  Daily for 3 days then every other day for 3-5 treatments.  If accelerated healing starts to slow or if you see no response, try modifying the time and frequency.  If increased time and frequency of 25% to 50% shows no benefit, try decreasing the treatments by 25% to 50% of the original protocol.

## ABSCESSES
Q1000 or Q100 Laser Placement:
Place a disposable glove on the laser, and then place the laser directly

over the abscess and any surrounding soft tissues that may be experiencing pain from the lesion.

Q1000: Mode 1 and Mode 3
Base Time: 3 minutes for each mode. (Range: 2 to 4 minutes) Use directly over the site of the abscess.
or:
Q100: Mode 1
Base Time: 9 minutes. (Range: 6 to 12 minutes) Use directly over the site of the abscess.

Use the 660 Enhancer for acupuncture or acupressure points.
Base Time: 1 minute. (Range: 1/2 to 2 minutes)

Use the 808 Enhancer directly over and around the lesion.
Base Time: 1 minute. (Range: 1/2 to 2 minutes)

Frequency of Use: Daily for 3 days, then every other day for 3-5 treatments, and then once weekly if needed. If accelerated healing starts to slow or if you see no response, try modifying the time and frequency. If increased time and frequency of 25% to 50% shows no benefit, try decreasing the treatments by 25% to 50% of the original protocol.


## ACUTE MOIST DERMATITIS/ HOT SPOTS
Q1000 or Q100 Laser Placement:
Place directly over the lesion and over any surrounding soft tissues that may be experiencing pain from the lesion.

Q1000: Mode 1 and Mode 3
Base Time: 2 minutes on each mode for each site. (Range: 1 to 3 minutes)
or:
Q100: Mode 1
Base Time: 6 minutes each site. (Range: 3 to 9 minutes)

Use 660 Enhancer for acupuncture or acupressure points and directly over and around the lesion.
Base Time: 1 minute each point and each site. (Range: 1/2 to 2 minutes)

or:
If the 660 Enhancer is not available, use 808 Enhancer directly over and around the lesion.
Base Time: 1/3 minute each site. (Range: 1/4 to 1/2 minute)

Frequency of Use: Daily for 3 days then every other day for 3-5 treatments. If accelerated healing starts to slow or if you see no response, try modifying the time and/or frequency of use. (Increase one or both by approximately 25%, and if that doesn't work, try decreasing by 25% from the original protocol.)


## ANAL GLAND INFLAMMATION
Q1000 or Q100 Laser Placement:
Place a disposable glove on the laser, and then place the laser directly over the inflammed area.

Q1000: Mode 1
Base Time: 2 minutes each site. (Range: 1 to 3 minutes)
or:
Q100: Mode 1
Base Time: 6 minutes each site. (Range: 3 to 9 minutes)

Use 660 Enhancer for acupuncture or acupressure points.
Base Time: 1 minute each point. (Range: 1/2 to 2 minutes)

Use 808 Enhancer over site of most severe pain on palpation.
Base Time: 2 minutes. (Range: 1 to 3 minutes)

Acute--Frequency of Use: Daily for 3-5 days, then every other day for 3 treatments, and then weekly if needed.
Chronic--Frequency of Use: Daily for 3 days, then every other day for 3 treatments, and then weekly or every two weeks as needed.


## BRONCHITIS
Q1000 or Q100 Laser Placement:
Apply the laser directly over ventral neck region where palpation elicits a cough.

Q1000:  Mode 1 and Mode 3
Base Time:  3 minutes each site. (Range:  2 to 4 minutes)
or:
Q100:  Mode 1
Base Time:  9 minutes each site. (Range:  6 to 12 minutes)

Use 660 Enhancer for acupuncture or acupressure points.
Base Time: 1 minute each point. (Range:  1/2 to 2 minutes)

Acute--Frequency of Use:  Daily for 3-5 days, then every other day for 3 treatments, and then weekly if needed.
Chronic--Frequency of Use:  Daily for 3-5 days, then every other day for 3 treatments, and then weekly to every two weeks as needed.

## BURNS
Q1000 or Q100 Laser Placement:
Place directly over the burn and over any surrounding soft tissues that may be experiencing contracture from the burn.

Q1000:  Mode 1 and Mode 3
Base Time:  3 minutes each site. (Range:  2 to 4 minutes)
or:
Q100:  Mode 1
Base Time:  9 minutes each site. (Range:  6 to 12 minutes)

Use 660 Enhancer for acupuncture or acupressure points or directly over more superficial burns.
Base Time: 1 minute. (Range:  1/2 to 2 minutes)

Use 808 Enhancer over deep burns.
Base Time: 2 minutes. (Range:  1 to 3 minutes)

Frequency of Use:  Twice daily for the first day, then daily for 7 days, then every other day for 3-5 treatments, and then every week as needed. If accelerated healing starts to slow or if you see no response, try modifying the time and frequency (plus or minus about 25%).

## CERVICAL OR NECK PAIN

Q1000 or Q100 Laser Placement:
Place directly over painful areas and over any surrounding tendons, ligaments, and muscles that are indirectly affected by the pain. (Target the origin and insertions of related muscles.)

Q1000: Mode 1 and Mode 3
Base Time: 2 minutes each site. (Range: 1 to 3 minutes)
or:
Q100: Mode 1
Base Time: 6 minutes each site. (Range: 3 to 9 minutes)

Use 660 Enhancer for acupuncture, acupressure, and trigger points.
Base Time: 1 minute each point. (Range: 1/2 to 2 minutes)

Use 808 Enhancer over site of most severe pain on palpation.
Base Time: 2 minutes each site. (Range: 1 to 3 minutes)

Acute--Frequency of Use: Daily for 5 days, then every other day for 3 treatments, and then weekly if needed.
Chronic--Frequency of Use: Daily for 3 days, then every other day for 3 treatments, and then weekly to every two weeks as needed.

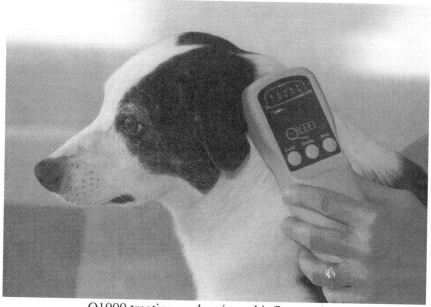

Q1000 treating neck pain and inflammation

**DECUBITAL ULCERS (Bed Sores)** – See Appendix for case study.
Q1000 or Q100 Laser Placement:
Place a disposable glove on the laser, and then place the laser directly over the ulcer and any surrounding soft tissues that may be experiencing contracture from the lesion. Remove the cause of the pressure creating the lesion. If the pet is debilitated, refer to the area of debilation and treat with the laser.

Q1000: Mode 1 and Mode 3
Base Time: 3 minutes each site. (Range: 2 to 4 minutes)
or:
Q100: Mode 1
Base Time: 9 minutes each site. (Range: 6 to 12 minutes)

Use 660 Enhancer for acupuncture or acupressure points.
Base Time: 1 minute each point. (Range: 1/2 to 2 minutes)

Use 808 Enhancer directly over and around lesion.
Base Time: 2 minutes each site. (Range: 1 to 3 minutes)

Frequency of Use: Daily for 3 days, then every other day for 3-5 treatments, and then once weekly if needed. If accelerated healing starts to slow or if you see no response, try modifying the time and frequency (plus or minus 25% to 50%).


**DEGENERATIVE MYELOPATHY**
Q1000 or Q100 Laser Placement:
Place directly over entire length of lumbar spine and epaxial muscles of the thoracic spine. Also place over atrophied muscles of rear quarters and over any painful joints.

Q1000: Mode 1 and Mode 3
Base Time: 3 minutes each site. (Range: 2 to 4 minutes)
or:
Q100: Mode 1
Base Time: 9 minutes each site. (Range: 6 to 12 minutes)

Use 660 Enhancer for acupuncture or acupressure points.
Base Time: 1 minute each site. (Range: 1/2 to 2 minutes)

Use 808 Enhancer over each lumbar vertebrae and on nerves exiting the spinal cord and on any areas where there is intense palpable pain.
Base Time: 2 minutes each site. (Range: 1 to 3 minutes)

Frequency of Use: Daily for 5 days, then every other day for 3 treatments, and then weekly.


**DENTAL PAIN**
Q1000 or Q100 Laser Placement:
Place directly over painful area or any soft tissues with inflammation. These lasers will not hurt enamel, dentin, or the pulp.

Q1000: Mode 1 and Mode 3
Base Time: 2 minutes each site. (Range: 1 to 3 minutes)
or:
Q100: Mode 1
Base Time: 6 minutes each site. (Range: 3 to 9 minutes)

Use 660 Enhancer over site of most severe pain and directly on the tooth if needed. Use on acupuncture or acupressure points.
Base Time: 1 minute each site and each point. (Range: 1/2 to 2 minutes)

Use 808 Enhancer over site of most severe pain and directly on the tooth if needed.
Base Time: 1 minute each site. (Range: 1/2 to 3 minutes)

Acute--Frequency of Use: Daily for 5 days, then every other day for 3 treatments, and then weekly if needed.
Chronic--Frequency of Use: Daily for 3 days, then every other day for 3 treatments, and then weekly or every two weeks as needed.


**EAR PAIN AND INFLAMMATION**
Q1000 or Q100 Laser Placement:
Place directly over the ear canal or ear flap where inflammation is present.

Q1000: For acute inflammation use Mode 1 and Mode 3.

33

For chronic inflammation, use Mode 1.
Base Time: 3 minutes each site. (Range: 2 to 4 minutes)
or:
Q100: Mode 1
Base Time: 9 minutes each site. (Range: 6 to 12 minutes)

Use 660 Enhancer for acupuncture or acupressure points.
Base Time: 1 minute each point. (Range: 1/2 to 2 minutes)

Use 808 Enhancer in ear canal or over site of most severe pain.
Base Time: 2 minutes each site. (Range: 1 to 3 minutes)

Acute--Frequency of Use: Daily for 3-5 days, then every other day for 3 treatments, and then weekly if needed.
Chronic--Frequency of Use: Daily for 3 days, then every other day for 3 treatments, and then weekly or every two weeks as needed. For hearing loss, aim the Q1000 or Q100 laser toward the middle and inner ear.

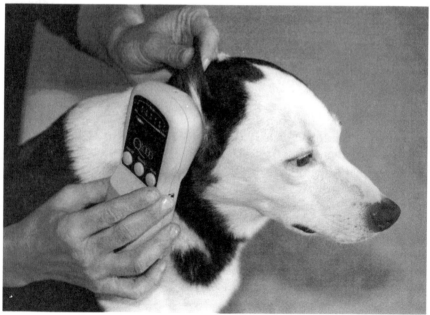

Q1000 treating ear pain and inflammation

## EOSINOPHILIC PLAQUES/ RODENT ULCERS

Q1000 or Q100 Laser Placement:
Place directly over the lesion and over any surrounding soft tissues that may be experiencing contracture from the lesion.

Q1000:  Mode 1 and Mode 3
Base Time: 3 minutes each site. (Range:  2 to 4 minutes)
or:
Q100:  Mode 1
Base Time:  9 minutes each site. (Range:  6 to 12 minutes)

Use 660 Enhancer for more superficial lesions.  Place directly over the lesion.
Base Time:  1 minute each site. (Range:  1/2 to 2 minutes)

Use 808 Enhancer for deep lesions.  Place directly over the lesion.
Base Time:  2 minutes each site. (Range:  1 to 3 minutes)

Frequency of Use:  Daily for 3-5 days, then every other day for 3-5 treatments, and then every week if needed.  If accelerated healing starts to slow or if you see no response, try modifying the time and frequency (plus or minus about 25% to 50%).


## HEAD TRAUMA

Q1000 or Q100 Laser Placement:
Cover the pet's eyes with a dry washcloth to help prevent the pet from looking directly at the laser. Treat directly over painful areas, and treat the entire skull as well, including the ligaments at the base of the skull.

Q1000:  Mode 2 and Mode 3
Base Time:  3 minutes each site. (Range:  2 to 4 minutes)
or:
Q100:  Mode 2
Base Time:  9 minutes each site. (Range:  6 to 12 minutes)

Use 660 Enhancer for acupuncture or acupressure points.
Base Time: 1 minute each site. (Range:  1/2 to 2 minutes)

Use 808 Enhancer over site of most severe pain on palpation.  Do not use on the eyes.

Base Time: 3 minutes each site. (Range: 2 to 4 minutes)

Frequency of Use: Daily for 5 days, and then every other day for 3 treatments, and then weekly if needed.

## INCISIONS
Q1000 or Q100 Laser Placement:
Place directly over the incision plus any surrounding soft tissues that may be experiencing pain from the lesion or possible contracture or tension.

Q1000: Mode 1 and 3
Base Time: 1.5 minutes each site. (Range: 1 to 2 minutes)
or:
Q100: Mode 1
Base Time: 4.5 minutes each site. (Range: 3 to 6 minutes)

Use 660 Enhancer for acupuncture or acupressure points and directly over and around the incision.
Base Time: 1 minute each point and each site. (Range: 1/2 to 2 minutes)
or:
Use 808 Enhancer directly over and around incision, if 660 Enhancer is not available.
Base Time: 1/3 minute each site. (Range: 1/4 to 1/2 minute)

Frequency of Use: Daily for 3 days, and then every other day for 3-5 treatments. If accelerated healing starts to slow or if you see no response, try modifying the time and frequency.

## JOINT PAIN AND INFLAMMATION (includes hip, shoulder, elbow, tarsus, carpus, etc.)
Q1000 or Q100 Laser Placement:
Place directly over painful area and over any surrounding tendons, ligaments, and muscles that are indirectly affected by the joint. (Target the origin and insertions of related muscles.)

Q1000:  Mode 1 and Mode 3
Base Time:  2 minutes each site.  (Range:  1 to 3 minutes)
or:
Q100:  Mode 1
Base Time:  6 minutes each site.  (Range:  3 to 9 minutes)

Use 660 Enhancer for acupuncture, acupressure, or trigger points.
Base Time:  1 minute each point.  (Range:  1/2 to 2 minutes)

Use 808 Enhancer over site of most severe pain on palpation.
Base Time:  3 minutes each site.  (Range:  2 to 4 minutes)

Acute--Frequency of Use:  Daily for 5 days, then every other day for
3 treatments, and then weekly if needed.
Chronic--Frequency of Use:  Daily for 3 days, then every other day for
3 treatments, and then weekly or every two weeks as needed.

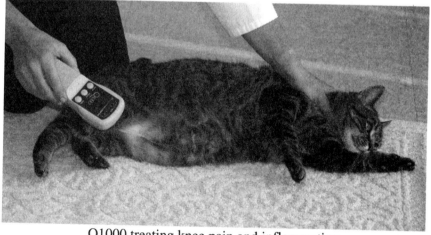

Q1000 treating knee pain and inflammation

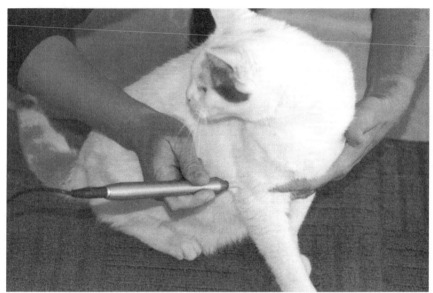
808 Enhancer treating elbow pain and inflammation

## LACERATIONS
Q1000 or Q100 Laser Placement:
Place directly over the laceration plus any surrounding soft tissues that may be experiencing pain from the lesion.

Q1000: Mode 1 and Mode 3
Base Time: 3 minutes over site. (Range: 2 to 4 minutes)
or:
Q100: Mode 1
Base Time: 9 minutes over site. (Range: 6 to 12 minutes)

Use 660 Enhancer for acupuncture or acupressure points.
Base Time: 1 minute each point. (Range: 1/2 to 2 minutes)

Use 808 Enhancer directly over and around lesion.
Base Time: 1 minute each site. (Range: 1/2 to 2 minutes)

Frequency of Use: Daily for 3 days, then every other day for 3-5 treatments, and then once weekly if needed. If accelerated healing starts to slow or if you see no response, try modifying the time and frequency.

## LICK GRANULOMAS

Q1000 or Q100 Laser Placement:
Place directly over the lesion plus any surrounding soft tissues that may be experiencing contracture from the lesion. Focus on treating the underlying cause creating the lesion. If the pet is licking because of pain, refer to the area of pain and treat with the laser.

Q1000:  Mode 1 and Mode 3
Base Time:  4 minutes over and around the lesion. (Range:  3 to 6 minutes)
or:
Q100:  Mode 1
Base Time:  12 minutes over and around the lesion. (Range:  9 to 18 minutes)

Use 660 Enhancer for acupuncture or acupressure points.
Base Time: 1 minute for each point. (Range:  1/2 to 2 minutes)

Use 808 Enhancer directly over and around lesion.
Base Time:  3 minutes each site. (Range:  2 to 4 minutes)

Frequency of Use:  Daily for 3-5 days, then every other day for 3-5 treatments, and then once weekly as needed.  If accelerated healing starts to slow or if you see no response, try modifying the time and frequency.


## LIMB PAIN AND INFLAMMATION

Q1000 or Q100 Laser Placement:
Place directly over painful area and over any surrounding tendons, ligaments, and muscles that are indirectly affected by the pain. Treat over the epaxial muscles (i.e., muscles along spine) that may be indirectly affected. SPECIAL NOTE:  Remember, forelimb pain can radiate from cervical pain.

Q1000:  Mode 1 and Mode 3
Base Time:  2 minutes each site. (Range:  1 to 3 minutes)
or:
Q100:  Mode 1
Base Time:  6 minutes each site. (Range:  3 to 9 minutes)

39

Use 660 Enhancer for acupuncture or acupressure points.
Base Time: 1 minute each point. (Range: 1/2 to 2 minutes)

Use 808 Enhancer over site of most severe pain on palpation.
Base Time: 2 minutes each site. (Range: 1 to 3 minutes)

Acute--Frequency of Use: Daily for 5 days, then every other day for 3 treatments, and then weekly if needed.
Chronic--Frequency of Use: Daily for 3 days, then every other day for 3 treatments, and then weekly or every two weeks as needed.


## LUMBAR PAIN AND INFLAMMATION
Q1000 or Q100 Laser Placement:
Place directly over painful areas plus any surrounding tendons, ligaments, and muscles that are indirectly affected by the pain. (Target the origin and insertions of related muscles.)

Q1000: Mode 1 and Mode 3
Base Time: 2 minutes each site. (Range: 1 to 3 minutes)
or:
Q100: Mode 1
Base Time: 6 minutes each site. (Range: 3 to 9 minutes)

Use 660 Enhancer for acupuncture, acupressure, and trigger points.
Base Time: 1 minute each point. (Range: 1/2 to 2 minutes)

Use 808 Enhancer over site of most severe pain on palpation.
Base Time: 2 minutes each site. (Range: 1 to 3 minutes)

Acute--Frequency of Use: Daily for 5 days, then every other day for 3 treatments, and then weekly if needed.
Chronic--Frequency of Use: Daily for 3 days, then every other day for 3 treatments, and then weekly to every two weeks as needed.


## MUSCLE PAIN AND INFLAMMATION
Q1000 or Q100 Laser Placement:
Place directly over painful area plus any surrounding tendons, ligaments, and muscles that are indirectly affected by the joint. (Target the origin and insertions of related muscles.)

Q1000:  Mode 1 and Mode 3
Base Time:  2 minutes each site.  (Range:  1 to 3 minutes)
or:
Q100:  Mode 1
Base Time:  6 minutes each site.  (Range:  3 to 9 minutes)

Use 660 Enhancer for acupuncture, acupressure, or trigger points.
Base Time: 1 minute each point.  (Range:  1/2 to 2 minutes)

Use 808 Enhancer over site of most severe pain on palpation.
Base Time:  3 minutes each site.  (Range:  2 to 4 minutes)

Acute--Frequency of Use:  Daily for 5 days, then every other day for 3 treatments, and then weekly if needed.
Chronic--Frequency of Use:  Daily for 3 days, then every other day for 3 treatments, and then weekly or every two weeks as needed.


## NERVE INJURY
Q1000 or Q100 Laser Placement:
Place directly over affected nerve and nerve root/plexus if applicable and over any surrounding tendons, ligaments, and muscles that are indirectly affected by the pain or condition.

Q1000:  Mode 1 and Mode 3
Base Time:  3 minutes each site.  (Range:  2 to 4 minutes)
or:
Q100:  Mode 1
Base Time:  9 minutes each site.  (Range:  6 to 12 minutes)

Use 660 Enhancer for acupuncture or acupressure points.
Base Time:  1 minute each point.  (Range:  1/2 to 2 minutes)

Use 808 Enhancer directly over the affected nerve and nerve root/ plexus.
Base Time:  3 minutes each site.  (Range:  2 to 4 minutes)

Acute--Frequency of Use:  Daily for 5 days, then every other day for 5 treatments, and then weekly until resolved.
Chronic--Frequency of Use:  Daily for 5 days, then every other day for 5 treatments, and then weekly to every two weeks as needed.

## POSTOPERATIVE PAIN SUPPORT

Q1000 or Q100 Laser Placement:
Place directly over surgical site during recovery plus any surrounding tissues that are indirectly affected by the pain.

Q1000:  Mode 1 and Mode 3
Base Time:  2 minutes each site. (Range:  1 to 3 minutes)
or:
Q100:  Mode 1
Base Time:  6 minutes each site. (Range:  3 to 9 minutes)

Use 660 Enhancer for acupuncture, acupressure, or trigger points.
Base Time: 1 minute each point. (Range:  1/2 to 2 minutes)

Use 808 Enhancer over site of most anticipated pain.
Base Time: 1 minute each site. (Range:  1/2 to 2 minutes)

Frequency of Use:  Daily for three days.  Also see the protocol for Incisions, page 36.

## PREOPERATIVE ANALGESIA

Q1000 or Q100 Laser Placement:
Prior to surgical scrubbing, place directly over surgical site and over any surrounding tissues that are indirectly affected by the pain.

Q1000:  Mode 1 and Mode 3
Base Time:  1 minute each site until entire area has been treated. (Range 1/2 to 2 minutes).
or:
Q100:  Mode 1
Base Time:  3 minutes each site until entire area has been treated. (Range 2 to 6 minutes).

Use 660 Enhancer for acupuncture, acupressure, or trigger points.
Base Time: 1 minute each point. (Range:  1/2 to 2 minutes)

Use 808 Enhancer over site of most anticipated pain.
Base Time:  1 minute each site. (Range:  1/2 to 2 minutes)

Frequency of Use:  Once prior to surgical scrubbing.

## PRIOR TO LOCAL ANESTHESIA
Q1000 or Q100 Laser Placement
Place directly over the site where the anesthesia will be used.

Q1000: Mode 1 and Mode 3
Base Time: 2 minutes each site. (Range: 1 to 3 minutes)
or:
Q100: Mode 1
Base Time: 6 minutes each site. (Range: 3 to 9 minutes)

Use 660 Enhancer directly over site.
Base Time: 2 minute each site. (Range: 1 to 3 minutes)
or:
Use 808 Enhancer directly over site, if 660 Enhancer is not available.
Base Time: 1/3 minute each site. (Range: 1/4 to 1/2 minute)

Frequency of Use: Once prior to administering local anesthesia.


## SACRAL OR TAIL PAIN AND INFLAMMATION
Q1000 or Q100 Laser Placement:
Place directly over painful areas and over any surrounding tendons, ligaments, and muscles that are indirectly affected by the pain. (Target the origin and insertions of related muscles.)

Q1000: Mode 1 and Mode 3
Base Time: 2 minutes each site. (Range: 1 to 3 minutes)
or:
Q100: Mode 1
Base Time: 6 minutes each site. (Range: 3 to 9 minutes)

Use 660 Enhancer for acupuncture, acupressure, and trigger points.
Base Time: 1 minute each point. (Range: 1/2 to 2 minutes)

Use 808 Enhancer over site of most severe pain on palpation.
Base Time: 2 minutes each site. (Range: 1 to 3 minutes)

Acute--Frequency of Use: Daily for 5 days, then every other day for 3 treatments, and then weekly if needed
Chronic--Frequency of Use: Daily for 3 days, then every other day for 3 treatments, and then weekly to every two weeks as needed.

## SCARRING

Q1000 or Q100 Laser Placement:
Place directly over the affected area and over surrounding soft tissues, such as skin and muscle, that may have been indirectly affected by contracture.

Q1000:  Mode 1 and Mode 3
Base Time:  3 minutes each site.  (Range:  2 to 4 minutes)
or:
Q100:  Mode 1
Base Time:  9 minutes each site.  (Range:  6 to 12 minutes)

Use 660 Enhancer for superficial scars, treating directly over the scar.
Base Time:  3 minutes each site.  (Range:  2 to 4 minutes)

Use 808 Enhancer for deep scars, treating directly over the scar and any surrounding area of palpable pain.
Base Time:  3 minutes each site.  (Range:  2 to 4 minutes)

Frequency of Use:  Daily for 5 days, then every other day for 3 treatments, and then weekly to every two weeks as needed.  If accelerated healing starts to slow or if you see no response, try modifying the time and frequency.


## SINUSITIS

Q1000 or Q100 Laser Placement:
Place a dry washcloth over the pet's eyes to help prevent the pet from looking into the laser.  Apply the laser directly over the affected sinus.

Q1000:  Mode 1 and Mode 3
Base Time:  3 minutes each site.  (Range:  2 to 4 minutes)
or:
Q100:  Mode 1
Base Time:  9 minutes each site.  (Range:  6 to 12 minutes)

Use 660 Enhancer over acupuncture or acupressure points.
Base Time:  1 minutes each point.  (Range:  1/2 to 2 minutes)

Use 808 Enhancer to treat over any swollen areas.
Base Time:  2 minutes each site.  (Range:  1 to 3 minutes)

Acute--Frequency of Use: Daily for 3-5 days, then every other day for 3 treatments, and then weekly if needed.
Chronic--Frequency of Use: Daily for 3-5 days, then every other day for 3 treatments, and then weekly to every two weeks as needed.

## THORACIC OR BACK PAIN
Q1000 or Q100 Laser Placement:
Place directly over painful areas and over any surrounding tendons, ligaments, and muscles that are indirectly affected by the pain. (Target the origin and insertions of related muscles.)

Q1000: Mode 1 and Mode 3
Base Time: 2 minutes each site. (Range: 1 to 3 minutes)
or:
Q100: Mode 1
Base Time: 6 minutes each site. (Range: 3 to 9 minutes)

Use 660 Enhancer for acupuncture, acupressure, or trigger points.
Base Time: 1 minute each point. (Range: 1/2 to 2 minutes)

Use 808 Enhancer over site of most severe pain on palpation.
Base Time: 2 minutes each site. (Range: 1 to 3 minutes)

Acute--Frequency of Use: Daily for 5 days, then every other day for 3 treatments, and then weekly if needed.
Chronic--Frequency of Use: Daily for 3 days, then every other day for 3 treatments, and then weekly or every two weeks as needed.

## TRIGGER POINT THERAPY
Q1000 or Q100 Laser Placement:
Place directly over palpated painful trigger points surrounding tendons, ligaments, and muscles that are indirectly affected by the pain.

Q1000: Mode 1 and Mode 3
Base Time: 3 minutes each site. (Range: 2 to 4 minutes)
or:

Q100:  Mode 1
Base Time:  9 minutes each site.  (Range:  6 to 12 minutes)

Use 660 Enhancer for trigger points.
Base Time:  1 minute for each trigger point.  (Range:  1/2 to 3 minutes)
or:
Use the 808 Enhancer directly over sites of most severe pain on palpation, if the 660 Enhancer is not available.
Base Time:  1/3 minute for each trigger point.  (Range:  1/4 to 1/2 minute)

Acute--Frequency of Use:  Daily for 2 days, then every other day for 2 treatments, and then weekly if needed.
Chronic--Frequency of Use:  Daily for 2 days, then every other day for 2 treatments, and then weekly or every two weeks as needed.


## VESTIBULAR DISEASE OR INNER EAR DISORDERS
Q1000 or Q100 Laser Placement:
Place the laser ventral to the ear, aiming toward the middle and inner ear.  If there is concurrent ear infection and inflammation, see the protocol for Ear Inflammation.  If the patient is a dog, remember to make sure that the pet is not hypothyroid.

Q1000:  Mode 2 and Mode 3
Base Time:  3 minutes each site.  (Range:  2 to 4 minutes)

Q100:  Mode 2
Base Time:  9 minutes each site.  (Range:  6 to 12 minutes)

Use 660 Enhancer for acupuncture or acupressure points.
Base Time:  1 minute each point.  (Range:  1/2 to 2 minutes)

Use 808 Enhancer directly over the bulla.
Base Time:  2 minutes.  (Range:  1 to 3 minutes)

Acute--Frequency of Use:  Daily for 3-5 days, then every other day for 3-5 treatments, and then weekly if needed.
Chronic--Frequency of Use:  Daily for 3 days, then every other day for 3 treatments, and then every two weeks as needed.

46

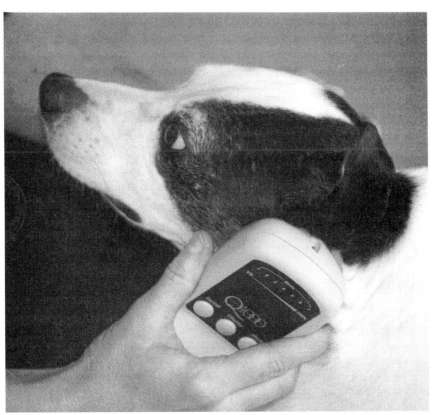

Q1000 treating the inner ear

# LOW-LEVEL LASER THERAPY FOR OTHER DISEASE PROCESSES

Because low-level laser works on the cellular level, in theory it can be applied to a variety of disease processes. In fact, there are many studies testing the efficacy of treating a variety of diseases with low-level laser therapy.

In the journal *Lasers in Surgery and Medicine*, de Castro e Silva, Zucoloto, Menegazzo, and others (2001), in a hepatic study in rats, showed a dramatic increase in mitochondrial activity after laser exposure and showed that the use of laser irradiation may promote a biostimulatory effect on early stages of liver regeneration.

Polosukhin (2000), in *Ultrastructure Pathology*, showed that endobronchiolar laser treatment of the lungs caused reversion of inflammation and stabilization of fibroblastic processes. Although additional research is needed, there may be considerable benefits from the use of low-level laser as an additional method of therapy for destructive lung diseases.

In *Lasers in Medical Science*, Guzzardella, Fini, Torricelli, and others (2002) showed that use of laser irradiation increased the percentage of healed area of bone defects in rats. The results suggest that low-level laser treatment may accelerate bone defect healing.

De Scheerder, Wang, Zhou, and others (2001), in *Journal of Clinical Laser Medicine and Surgery*, showed that low-level laser treatments may reduce angiographic in-stent restenosis and neointimal hyperplasia in porcine models of coronary stent implantation.

Because there is no evidence of any adverse reactions in pets associated with use of low-level laser therapy, I treat my own pets with low-level laser therapy for virtually anything and everything that ails them. The general protocol that I use for my pet's internal and metabolic diseases and conditions includes:

1. Use the Q1000 on Mode 3.
2. Apply directly over the origin of the disorder.
3. Apply to the area for 3 minutes.
4. Use daily for 3 days, then every other day for 3 treatments, and then once weekly if needed.

48

# TRIGGER POINT THERAPY USING LOW-LEVEL LASER

Trigger points are painful areas located in muscles or fascia that, with careful examination, will palpate as hard nodules of various size. There are predictable locations to look for these trigger points. (Some of them correspond to acupuncture points.) The low-level laser is an excellent device to treat these areas because of the relatively brief time it takes to treat a trigger point with a laser compared to massage and other forms of trigger-point stimulation. (Teaching trigger-point therapy is beyond the scope of this book, but this book does include protocols for trigger-point therapy for those veterinarians who do have some knowledge of trigger points.)

Trigger points that are painful may be responsible for the pain associated with some lamenesses. For example, a nodule in a pet's leg may prevent full lengthening of the muscle, resulting in weakening of the leg. Referred pain and cellular changes may also result from the trigger point. Once the trigger point is treated, the associated pain or lameness improves.

See pages 45-46 for trigger point protocol.

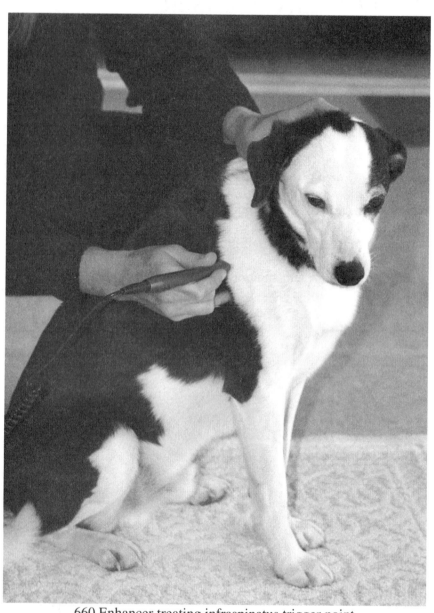

660 Enhancer treating infraspinatus trigger point

# ACUPUNCTURE USING LOW-LEVEL LASER

Low-level laser is an effective way to stimulate acupuncture points. It can replace acupuncture needle stimulation, therefore making laser stimulation a good option for children and other sensitive individuals.

Schlager, Offer, and Baldissera (1998), in the *British Journal of Anesthesia*, showed that laser acupuncture with wavelengths of 670 nanometers at 10 milliwatts reduced postoperative vomiting in children undergoing strabismus eye surgery. The placebo control group had an 85% incidence versus 25% in the laser-treated group.

In *Medicinski Pregled*, Milojevic and Kuruc (2003) showed that laser acupuncture treatment of patients with bronchial asthma may improve lung function and gas exchange parameters. Also, patients undergoing successive treatments showed prolonged periods of remission and decreased severity of asthmatic attacks.

The use of low-level laser to stimulate acupuncture points in pets may be benenficial in several ways. Compared to traditional acupunture, the low-level laser is more comfortable for the pets and takes less time. In addition, there are fewer complications because there is no risk of bleeding, infection or accidental insertion of a needle in the wrong place. Finally, low-level laser is considerably easier to use because the device is simply placed over a point, whereas traditional acupuncture requires insertion of a needle to a specific depth, which can vary depending upon the location and the condition being treated.

Stimulation of acupuncture points in the ear is a common method of acupuncture treatment for a variety of ailments, but acupuncture in a pet's ear can be problematic because of the complications associated with bleeding and the potential for ear hematomas. With the use of low-level laser, however, ear acupuncture points can be stimulated without the fear of these complications.

In practice, low-level laser can be used on acupuncture points to help treat a variety of ailments, including pain, liver disorders, gastritis, and pruritus. There are many point prescriptions, for pain and other ailments in pets, that employ use of the low-level laser instead of needles.

To better understand the complexities of acupuncture, please consult an acupuncture professional. Teaching acupuncture is beyond the scope of this book, but this book does include acupuncture-point low-level laser protocols for those veterinarians who do have some knowledge of acupuncture.

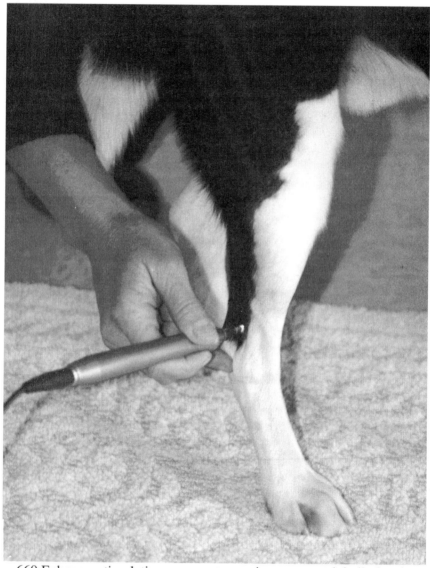

660 Enhancer stimulating acupuncture point to treat pelvic limb pain

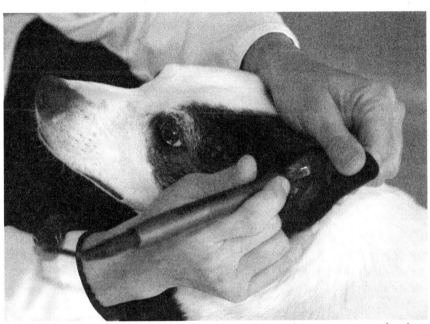

660 Enhancer stimulating an ear acupuncture point to treat sacral pain

# FAILURE TO RESPOND TO LOW-LEVEL LASER

As veterinarians, we strive to provide our pets with the opportunity to be as pain free as possible and to have the best possible recoveries. In our efforts to accomplish this goal, we use a multimodal approach to treatments, combining the best available therapies in the best ways possible. However, sometimes our most skillful and diligent efforts fail to produce all of the desired results. If you use low-level laser therapy as part of your multimodal approach to veterinary medicine and do not get the results that you hope for, consider the following as possible reasons for disappointing results:

Reasons for Treatment Failure
1. Reinjury of area
2. Not applying the laser at the appropriate site
3. Administering treatments for periods of time that are too long
4. Administering treatments for periods of time that are too short
5. Administering treatments too frequently
6. Administering treatments too infrequently
7. Not using the proper laser mode
8. Improper nutrition during recovery
9. Not utilizing other forms of therapy along with low-level laser
10. Another disease condition complicating the recovery

# APPENDIX

## CASE STUDY – Decubital ulcer (bed sore) treated with low-level laser therapy as part of a multimodal approach to treatment

Kody was a 15-year-old neutered male Samoyed debilitated with paralysis from degenerative myelopathy. He struggled with an 8 x 2 cm deep, nonhealing decubital ulcer (bed sore) over his right hip. The standard treatment for a decubital ulcer is to reduce pressure over the area and use a combination of antibiotics, an anti-inflammatory and rigorous hygiene. The realistic goal of this combination of therapies is not to provide a cure, but rather to keep the ulcer form getting any worse. Typically lesions like this in debilitated pets worsen and do not heal. With Kody, I used an oral antibiotic, a topical antibiotic, an anti-inflammatory, and rigorous hygiene. In addition to this standard treatment, however, I also used a combination of local oxygen therapy and low-level laser therapy. (I used the decubital ulcer low-level laser therapy protocol that is specified in this book.) The results are shown in the photographs: The lesion healed completely within a period of eight weeks.

Because I used a multimodal approach (and because this was not a scientific study with a control group) I suppose that I can't really say for sure that the cure was the result of the low-level laser. And even if the ulcer was cured by the laser, individual results will vary, and I don't know that my result was a typical result. What I do know, however, is that I used the low-level laser as part of a multimodal approach to treat a bad situation that usually gets worse, and I ended up with a miraculous cure--and that's good enough for me. You can bet I'll use the low-level laser next time in the same way for the same situation.

The photographs that follow on the next three pages were taken over a period of eight weeks:

57

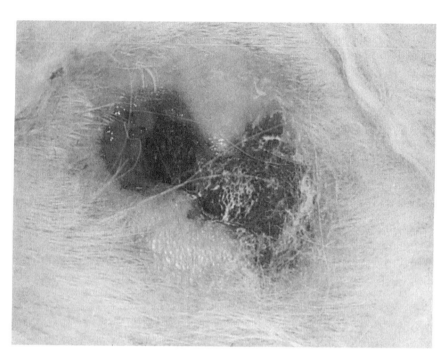

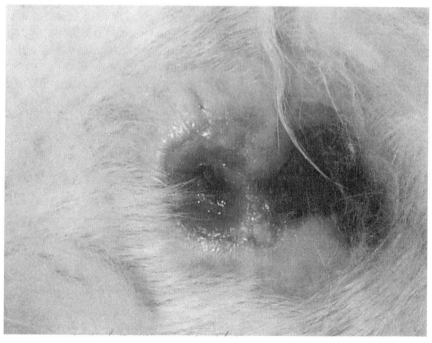

58

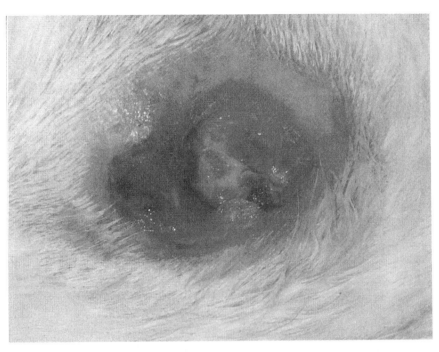

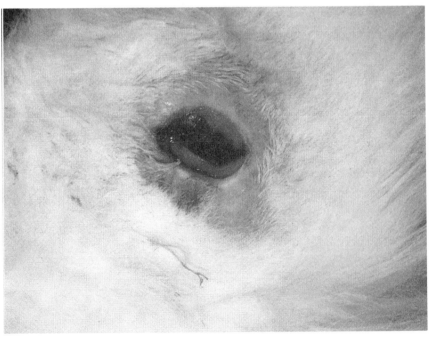

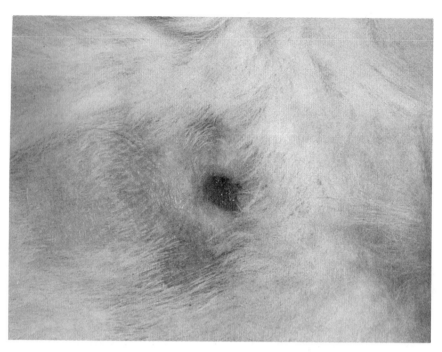

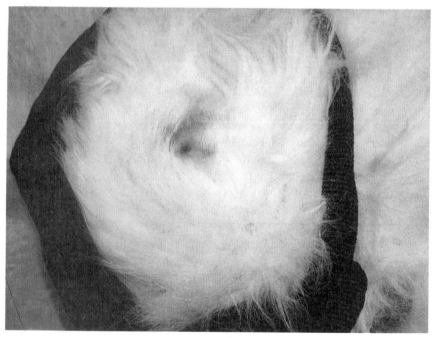

60

# REFERENCE LIST

Ailioaie, C., and L. Ailioaie. 2000. Treatment of bronchial asthma with low-level laser in attack-free period at children. *Proceedings of SPIE* 4166: 303-308.

Akai, M., M. Usuba, T. Maeshima, Y. Shirasaki, and S. Yasuoka. 1997. Laser's effect on bone and cartilage change induced by joint immobilization: An experiment with animal model. *Lasers in Surgery and Medicine* 21, no. 5: 480-484.

Almeida-Lopes, L., J. Rigau, R. A. Zangaro, J. Guidugli-Neto, and M. M. Jaeger. 2001. Comparison of the low level laser therapy effects on cultured human gingival fibroblasts proliferation using different irradiance and same fluence. *Lasers in Surgery and Medicine* 29, no. 2: 179-184.

Almeida-Lopes, L., M. M. Jaeger, A. Brugnera Jr., and J. Rigau. 1998. Action of low-power laser irradiation on the proliferation of human gingival fibroblasts in vitro. *Proceedings of SPIE* 3248: 156-161.

Amaral, A. C., N. A. Parizotto, and T. F. Salvini. 1998. He-Ne laser action in the regeneration of the tibialis anterior muscle of mice. *Proceedings of the 2nd Congress of the World Association for Laser Therapy, Kansas City*: 18-19.

Amaral, A. C., N. A. Parizotto, and T. F. Salvini. 2001. Dose-dependency of low-energy HeNe laser effect in regeneration of skeletal muscle in mice. *Lasers in Medical Science* 16, no. 1: 44-51.

American Society for Laser Medicine and Surgery. 1999. American Society for Laser Medicine and Surgery 19th annual meeting, Lake Buena Vista, Florida, USA, April 16-18, 1999. Abstracts. *Lasers in Surgery and Medicine* Supplement 11: 1-78.

Ananchenko, V. G., A. G. Khanin, and O. V. Gostishcheva. 1999. [Cytological parameters of bronchoalveolar lavage in patients with chronic obstructive bronchitis exposed to laser radiation of blood.] *Terapevticheskii arkhiv* 71, no. 11: 65-67.

Asagai, Y., T. Ueno, and T. Ohshiro. 1998. Application of low reactive-level laser therapy (LLLT) in the functional training of cerebral palsy patients. *Proceedings of the 2nd Congress of the World Association for Laser Therapy, Kansas City*: 99-100.

Asagai, Y. A. Imakire, and T. Ohshiro. 2000-2001. Thermographic effects of laser therapy in patients with cerebral palsy. Abstract. Millennium edition, *Journal of Laser Therapy* 12.

Asagai, Y., A. Imakire, and T. Ohshiro. 2000-2001. Thermographic study of low level laser therapy for acute-phase injury. Abstract. Millennium edition, *Journal of Laser Therapy* 12.

Balakirev, S. A., L. I. Gusev, M. B. Kazanova, M. V. Kiselevskii, and A. Ia. Grabovshchiner. 2000. [Low-intensity laser therapy in pediatric oncology.] *Voprosy Onkologii* 46, no. 4: 459-461.

Barasch, A., D. E. Peterson, J. M. Tanzer, J. A. D'Ambrosio, K. Nuki, M. M. Schubert, et al. 1995. Helium-neon laser effects on conditioning-induced oral mucositis in bone marrow transplantation patients. *Cancer* 76, no. 12: 2550-2556.

Baratto, L., R. Capra, M. Farinelli, P. Monteforte, P. Morasso and G. Rovetta. 2000. A new type of very low-power modulated laser: Soft-tissue changes induced in osteoarthritic patients revealed by sonography. *International Journal of Clinical Pharmacology Research* 20, nos. 1-2: 13-16.

Barber, A., J. E. Lugar, A. Karpf, Kh. Salame, B. Shlomi, G. Kogan, et al. 2000-2001. Advances in laser therapy for bone repair. Abstract. Millennium edition, *Journal of Laser Therapy* 13.

Basford, J. R., C. G. Sheffield, and W. S. Harmsen. 1999. Laser therapy: A randomized, controlled trial of the effects of low-intensity Nd:YAG laser irradiation on musculoskeletal back pain. *Archives of Physical Medicine and Rehabilitation* 80, no. 6: 647-652.

Ben-Dov N., G. Shefer, A. Irintchev, A. Wernig, U. Oron, and O. Halevy. 1999. Low-energy laser irradiation affects satellite cell proliferation and differentiation in vitro. *Biochimica et Biophysica Acta* 1448, no. 3: 372-80.

Bensadoun, R. J. 2002. Low-level laser therapy: A real hope in the management of chemo-induced and radiation-induced mucositis? *Cancer Journal* 8, no. 3: 236-238.

Beyer, W., R. Baumgartner, and S. Tauber. 1998. Dosimetric analysis for low-level laser therapy (LLLT) of the human inner ear at 593 nm and 633 nm. *Proceedings of SPIE* 3569: 56-59.

Bisht, D., R. Mehrotra, P. A. Singh, S. C. Atri, and A. Kumar. 1999. Effect of helium-neon laser on wound healing. *Indian Journal of Experimental Biology* 37, no. 2: 187-189.

Bjordal, J. M., C. Couppé, R. T. Chow, J. Tunér, and E. A. Ljunggren. 2003. A systematic review of low level laser therapy with location-specific doses for pain from chronic joint disorders. *The Australian Journal of Physiotherapy* 49, no. 2: 107-116.

Blood, D. C., and Virginia P. Studdert. 1988. *Baillière's Comprehensive Veterinary Dictionary*. London: Bailliére Tindall.

Bonis, B., L. Kemeny, A. Dobozy, Z. Bor, G. Szabo, and F. Ignacz. 1997. 308 nm UVB excimer laser for psoriasis. Abstract. *Lancet* 350, no. 9090: 1522.

Brugnera Jr., A., A. E. Garrini, A. Pinheiro, D. H. Souza Campos, E. Donamaria, F. Magalhães, et al. 2000-2001. Laser therapy in the treatment of dental hypersensitivity: A histologic study and clinical application. Abstract. Millennium edition, *Journal of Laser Therapy* 12.

Brugnera Jr., A., F. M. Cruz, F. A. Zanin, and J. D. Pecora. 1999. Clinical results evaluation of dentinary hypersensitivity patients treated with laser therapy. *Proceedings of SPIE* 3593: 66-68.

Chor, A., A. B. Sotero Caio, A. Mello de Azevedo. 2001. The irreplaceable image: Amelioration of oral mucosal lesions of acute graft-versus-host disease by low-level laser therapy. *Haematologica* 86, no. 12: 1321.

Cohen, N., R. Lubart, S. Rubinstein, and H. Breitbart. 1998. Light irradiation of mouse spermatozoa: Stimulation of in vitro fertilization and calcium signals. *Photochemistry and Photobiology* 68, no. 3: 407-413.

de Castro e Silva Jr., O., S. Zucoloto, L. A. Menegazzo, R. G. Granato, L. G. Marcassa, and V. S. Bagnato. 2001. Laser enhancement in hepatic regeneration for partially hepatectomized rats. *Lasers in Surgery and Medicine* 29, no. 1: 73-77.

de Paula Eduardo, C., and S. Gouw-Soares. 2001. The use of lasers for endodontic applications in dentistry. *Medical Laser Application* 16, no. 3: 231-243.

De Scheerder, I. K., K. Wang, X. R. Zhou, M. Szilard, E. Verbeken, Q. B. Ping, et al. 2001. Optimal dosing of intravascular low-power red laser light as an adjunct to coronary stent implementation: Insights from a porcine coronary stent model. *Journal of Clinical Laser Medicine and Surgery* 19, no. 5: 261-265.

Enwemeka, C. S., and G. K. Reddy. 2000-2001. The biological effects of laser therapy and other physical modalities on connective tissue repair processes. Abstract. Millennium edition, *Journal of Laser Therapy* 12.

Friedmann, H., R. Lubart, I. Laulicht, and S. Rochkind. 1991. A possible explanation of laser-induced stimulation and damage of cell cultures. *Journal of Photochemistry and Photobiology, B: Biology* 11, no. 1: 87-91.

Gasparyan, L., and S. Grigoryan. 1998. Low level laser therapy of genital tract chronic inflammations. *Proceedings of the 2nd Congress of the World Association for Laser Therapy, Kansas City*: 82-83.

Gruszka, M., W. Amryn, R. Fiszerman, J. Pucineri, A. Soerensen, and O. M. Noguera. 1998. Effect of low energy laser therapy on herniated lumbar discs. Abstract. *Lasers in Surgery and Medicine* Supplment 10, abstract 25: 6.

Grzesiak-Janas, G., and A. Janas. 2001. Conservative closure of antro-oral communication stimulated with laser light. *Journal of Clinical Laser Medicine and Surgery* 19, no. 4: 181-184.

Guzzardella, G. A., D. Tigani, P. Torricelli, M. Fini, L. Martini, G. Morrone, et al. 2001. Low-power diode laser stimulation of surgical osteochondral defects: Results after 24 weeks. *Artificial Cells, Blood Substitutes, and Immobilization Biotechnology* 29, no. 3: 235-44.

Guzzardella, G. A., M. Fini, P. Torricelli, G. Giavaresi, and R. Giardino. 2002. Laser stimulation on bone defect healing: an in vitro study. *Lasers in Medical Science* 17, no. 3: 216-220.

Hode, L., and J. Tunér. 2000. Low-level laser therapy (LLLT) versus light-emitting diode therapy (LEDT): What is the difference? *Proceedings of SPIE* 4166: 90-97.

Idrisova, L. T., D. A. Enikeev, and T. V. Vasil'eva. 2000. [The effect of intravenous laser irradiation of the blood on the brain bioelectrical activity in patients in the postcomatose period.] *Voprosy Kurortologii, Fizioterapii, I Lechebnoi Fizicheskoi Kultury* 2: 28-31.

Ilich-Stoianovich, O., E. L. Nasonov, and R. M. Balabanova. 2000. [Effects of low-intensity infrared impulse laser therapy on inflammation activity markers in patients with rheumatoid arthritis.] *Terapevticheskii arkhiv.* 72, no. 5: 32-34.

Itoh, T., H. Murakami, K. Orihashi, T. Sueda, Y. Kusumoto, M. Kakehashi, et al. 2000. Low power laser protects human erythrocytes in an in vitro model of artificial heart-lung machines. *Artificial Organs* 24, no. 11: 870-873.

Karu, T. I., N. I. Afanasyeva, S. F. Kolyakov, L. V. Pyatibrat, and L. Welser. 2001. Changes in absorbance of monolayer of living cells induced by laser radiation at 633, 670 and 820 nm. *IEEE Journal of Selected Topics in Quantum Electronics* 7, no. 6: 982-988.

Katsuyama, I., T. Hashimoto, Y. Ohta, H. Otsuka, and O. Kemmotsu. 1998. Laser irradiation suppresses hyperalgesia in neuropathic rats. *Proceedings of the 2nd Congress of the World Association for Laser Therapy, Kansas City*: 28.

Kjusephashova, Ts. and I. Haydouchka. 1997. Laser therapy and immunostimulators in patients with acute orofacial infections. Abstract. *Abstracts of ICMART '97 International Medical Acupuncture Symposium*: 79.

Kobayashi, M., H. Matsuoka, and J. Kubota. 1998. Studies of the diode laser therapy on blood supply in the rat model. *Proceedings of the 2nd Congress of the World Association for Laser Therapy, Kansas City*: 70-71.

Korolev, Iu. N., L. N. Panova, and M. S. Geniatulina. 2000. [The correction of the subcellular postradiation changes in the hypothalamus and parathyroid gland by using low-intensity laser radiation (an experimental study).] *Voprosy Kurortologii, Fizioterapii, I Lechebnoi Fizicheskoi Kultury* 3: 3-4.

Kovalyova, T. V. 1999. Clinical-pathogenetical aspects of combined laser therapy efficient use in patients with diabetes mellitus, as compared with pharmacologic therapy. Abstract. *Proceedings of 2nd International Congress "Laser and Health '99"*: 365.

Kovalyova T.V., A. V. Farvayeva, L. T. Pimenov, and S. M. Denisov. 1999. Dynamics of hyperlipidemia and peripheral blood flow in patients with diabetes mellitus after the course of combined laser therapy in conditions of out-patient department. Abstract. *Proceedings of 2nd International Congress "Laser and Health '99"*: 313.

Kovalyova, T. V., and L. T. Pimenov. 1999. Dynamics of lipid metabolism and peripheral blood flow rates in patients with atherosclerosis associated with with renal pathology after the course of combined laser therapy. Abstract. *Proceedings of 2nd International Congress "Laser and Health '99"*: 311.

Kreisler, M., A. B. Christoffers, B. Willershausen, and B. d'Hoedt. 2003. Effect of low-level GaAlAs laser irradiation on the proliferation rate of human periodontal ligament fibroblasts: An in vitro study. *Journal of Clinical Periodontology* 30, no. 4: 353-358.

Kreisler, M. B., H. A. Haj, N. Noroozi, and B. Willershausen. 2004. Efficacy of low level laser therapy in reducing postoperative pain after endodontic surgery – a randomized double blind clinical study. *International Journal of Oral and Maxillofacial Surgery* 33, no. 1: 38-41.

Kubota, J. 2002. Effects of diode laser therapy on blood flow in axial pattern flaps in the rat model. *Lasers in Medical Science* 17, no. 3: 146-153.

Kurumada, F. 2000-2001. [A study of the application of Ga-As semiconductor laser to endodontics. The effect of laser irradiation on the activation of inflammatory cells and the vital pulpotomy.] *Ou Daigaku Shigakushi* 17 (1990): 233-244.

Lagan, K. M., S. M. McDonough, B. A. Clements, and G. D. Baxter. 2000. A case report of low intensity laser therapy (LILT) in the management of venous ulceration: Potential effects of wound debridement upon efficacy. *Journal of Clinical Laser Medicine & Surgery* 18, no. 1: 15-22.

Lichtenstein, D., and B. Morag. 1998. Laser therapy in ambulatory patients with venous stasis ulcers. *Proceedings of the 2nd Congress of the World Association for Laser Therapy, Kansas City*: 31-32.

Lizarelli, R. F., T. L. Lamano-Carvalho, and L. G. Brentegani. 1999. Histometric evaluation of the healing of the dental alveolus in rats after irradiation with a low-powered GaAlAs laser. *Proceedings of SPIE* 3593: 49-56.

Longo, L., Z. Simunovic, M. Postiglione, and M. Postiglione. 1997. Laser therapy for fibromyositic rheumatisms. *Journal of Clinical Laser Medicine and Surgery* 15, no. 5: 217-220.

Lubart, R., H. Friedmann, N. Grossman, N. Cohen, and H. Breitbart. 1997. Reactive oxygen species and photobiostimulation. *Proceedings of SPIE* 3198: 12-18.

Lubart, R., H. Friedmann, M. Sinyakov, N. Cohen, and H. Breitbart. 1997. Changes in calcium transport in mammalian sperm mitochondria and plasma membranes caused by 780 nm irradiation. *Lasers in Surgery and Medicine* 21, no. 5: 493-499.

Luger, E. J., S. Rochkind, Y. Wollman, G. Kogan, and S. Dekel. 1998. Effect of low-power laser irradiation on the mechancal properties of bone fracture healing in rats. *Lasers in Surgery and Medicine* 22, no. 2: 97-102.

Lytle, Larry. 2003. *Low Level Laser User's Manual*. Portland, OR: Wowapi, Inc.

Marks, R., and F. de Palma. 1999. Clinical efficacy of low power laser therapy in osteoarthritis. *Physiotherapy Research International* 4, no. 2: 141-157.

Mijailovic, B., D. Karadaglic, T. Mladenovic, L. Popovic, R. D. Zecevic, and M. D. Pavlovic. 2001. Painful piezogenic pedal papules – successful low level laser therapy. *Acta Dermatovenerologica Alpina, Pannonica et Adriatica* 10, no. 3.

Mikhailov, V. A., O. A. Alexandrova, and I. N. Denisov. 2000. Use of the immunomodulative influence of low-level laser radiation in the treatment of an autoimmune thyroiditis. *Proceedings of SPIE* 4166: 319-322.

Milojevic, M., and V. Kuruc. 2003. [Low power laser biostimulation in the treatment of bronchial asthma.] *Medicinski Pregled* 56, no. 9-10: 413-418.

Miloro, M., and M. Repasky. 2000. Low-level laser effect on neurosensory recovery after sagittal ramus osteomy. *Oral Surgery, Oral Medicine, Oral Pathology, Oral Radiology, and Endodontics* 89, no. 1: 12-18.

Morrone, G., G. A. Guzzardella, D. Tigani, P. Torricelli, M. Fini, and R. Giardino. 2000. Biostimulation of human chondrocytes with Ga-Al-As diode laser: 'In vitro' research. *Artificial Cells, Blood Substitutes, and Immobilization Biotechnology* 28, no. 2: 193-201.

Morrone, G., G. A. Guzzardella, P. Torricelli, M. Rocca, D. Tigani, G. B. Brodano, et al. 2000. Osteochondral lesion repair of the knee in the rabbit after low-power diode Ga-Al-As laser biostimulation: An experimental study. *Artificial Cells, Blood Substitutes, and Immobilization Biotechnology* 28, no. 4: 321-336.

Navtrátil, L., and B. Navtrátilová. 2000. Possibilities of the treatment of certain diseases in stomatology with the help of non-invasive laser therapy. *Proceedings of SPIE* 4166: 273-279.

Nelson, A. J., and M. H. Friedman. 2000-2001. Somatosensory trigeminal evoked potential amplitudes following low level laser and sham irradiation over time. Abstract. Millennium edition, *Journal of Laser Therapy* 13.

Nikolic, B. 1997. Application of laser acupuncture in the treatment of periarthritis humeroscapularis. Abstract. *Abstracts of ICMART '97 International Medical Acupuncture Symposium*: 55.

Nikolic, S., and Z. Trojacanec. 1997. Low energy laser in the treatment of low back pain. Abstract. *Abstracts of ICMART '97 International Medical Acupuncture Symposium*: 91.

Nussbaum, E. L. 1999. Low-intensity laser therapy for benign fibrotic lumps in the breast following reduction mammaplasty. *Physical Therapy* 79, no. 7: 691-698.

Oasevich, I. A., and A. G. Shargorodskii. 1999. [Low-intensity infrared laser radiation in the diagnosis and combined treatment of acute nonspecific lymphadenitis of the face and neck in children.] *Stomatologiia* 78, no. 2: 28-30.

Ohno, T. 1997. [Pain suppressive effect of low power laser irradiation: A quantitative analysis of substance P in the rat spinal dorsal root ganglion.] *Nippon Ika Daigaku Zasshi* 64, no. 5: 395-400.

Ozdemir, F., M. Birtane, and S. Kokino. 2001. The clinical efficacy of low-power laser therapy on pain and function in cervical osteoarthritis. *Clinical Rheumatology* 20, no. 3: 181-184.

Parizotto, N. A., and V. Baranauskas. 1998. Structural analysis of collagen fibrils after He-Ne laser photostimulation of regenerating rat tendon. *Proceedings of the 2nd Congress of the World Association for Laser Therapy, Kansas City*: 66.

Passeniouk, A. N., and V. A. Mikhailov. 2000. Application of the low-level laser therapy for the treatment of vaginitis. *Proceedings of SPIE* 4166: 316-318.

Pinheiro, A. L., E. T. Cavalcanti, T. I. Pinheiro, M. J. Alves, E. R. Miranda, A. S. De Quevedo, et al. 1998. Low-level laser therapy is an important tool to treat disorders of the maxillofacial region. *Journal of Clinical Laser Medicine and Surgery* 16, no. 4: 223-226.

Pinheiro, A. L. B., M. G. Oliveira, P. P. M. Martins, L. M. Pedreira Ramalho, M. A. Matos de Oliveira, A. Novaes Júnior, and R. Amadei Nicolau. 2000-2001. Biomodulatory effects of LLLT on bone regeneration. Abstract. Millennium edition, *Journal of Laser Therapy* 13.

Poliakova, A. G., N. D. Gladkova, and T. D. Triphonova. 1997. Laserpuncture in patients with rheumatoids arthritis. Abstract. *Abstracts of ICMART '97 International Medical Acupuncture Symposium*: 52.

Polosukhin, V. V. 2000. Ultrastructure of the blood and lymphatic capillaries of the respiratory tissue during inflammation and endobronchial laser therapy. *Ultrastructural Pathology* 24, no. 3: 183-189.

Pöntinen, P. J. 2002. Laseracupuncture. *Proceedings of the 4th Congress of the World Association for Laser Therapy*: 111-116.

Pöntinen, P. J. 1992. *Low Level Laser Therapy as a Medical Treatment Modality*. Tampere, Finland. Art Urpo Ltd.

Prokof'eva, G. L., E. V. Kravchenko, V. P. Mozherenkov, S. G. Sergushev, and A. Iu. Balarev. 1996. [Effects of low-intensity infrared laser irradiation on the eye (an experimental study).] *Vestnik Oftalmologii* 112, no. 1: 31-32.

Reddy, G. K., L. Stehno-Bittel, and C. S. Enwemeka. 2001. Laser photostimulation accelerates wound healing in diabetic rats. *Wound Repair and Regeneration* 9, no. 3: 248-255.

Rochkind, S., A. Shahar, M. Alon, and Z. Nevo. 2002. Transplantation of embryonal spinal cord nerve cells cultured on biodegradable microcarriers followed by low power laser irradiation for the treatment of traumatic paraplegia in rats. *Neurological Research* 24, no. 4: 355-360.

Rochkind, S., M. Nissan, M. Alon, M. Shamir, and K. Salame. 2001. Effects of laser irradiation on the spinal cord for the regeneration of crushed peripheral nerve in rats. *Lasers in Surgery and Medicine* 28, no. 3: 216-219.

Samoilova, K., and S. Snopov. 1998. A key role on whole circulating blood modification in therapeutic effects of ultraviolet and visible light. *Proceedings of the 2nd Congress of the World Association for Laser Therapy, Kansas City*: 92-94.

Samoilova, K. A., O. I. Zubanova, S. A. Snopov, N. A. Mukhuradze, and V. M. Mikhelson. 1998. Single skin exposure to visible polarized light induces rapid modification of entire circulating blood. *Proceedings of SPIE* 3569: 26-33.

Sasaki, K., T. Ohshiro, S. Yasuda, Ta. Ohshiro, K. Yamamoto, and K. Inoue. 1998. Lower level laser therapy (LLLT) for thromboangitis obliterans. *Proceedings of the 2nd Congress of the World Association for Laser Therapy, Kansas City*: 95-96.

Schaffer, M., H. Bonel, R. Sroka, P. M. Schaffer, M. Busch, H. Sittek, et al. 2000. Magnetic resonance imaging (MRI) controlled outcome of side effects caused by ionizing radiation, treated with 780 nm-diode laser – preliminary results. *Journal of Photochemistry and Photobiology, B: Biology* 59, nos. 1-3: 1-8.

Schaffer, M., H. Bonel, R. Sroka, P. M. Schaffer, M. Busch, M. Reiser, et al. 2000. Effects of 780 nm diode laser irradiation on blood microcirculation: Preliminary findings on time-dependent T1-weighted contrast-enhanced magnetic resonance imaging (MRI). *Journal of Photochemistry and Photobiology, B: Biology* 54, no. 1: 55-60.

Schaffer, M., R. Sroka, C. Fuchs, U. Schrader-Reichardt, P. M. Schaffer, M. Busch, et al. 1997. Biomodulative effects induced by 805 nm laser light irradiation of normal and tumor cells. *Journal of Photochemistry and Photobiology, B: Biology* 40: 253-257.

Schindl, A., and R. Neumann. 1999. Low-intensity laser therapy is an effective treatment for recurrent herpes simplex infection. Results from a randomized double-blind placebo-controlled study. *The Journal of Investigative Dermatology* 113, no. 2: 221-223.

Schindl, A., M. Schindl, H. Pernerstorfer-Schoen, and L. Schindl. 2000. Low-intensity laser therapy: A review. *Journal of Investigative Medicine* 48, no. 5: 312-326.

Schindl, A., M. Schindl, L. Schindl, W. Jurecka, H. Hönigsmann, and F. Breier. 1998. Increased dermal neovascularization after low dose laser therapy of a chronic radiation ulcer determined by a video measuring system. *Proceedings of the 2nd Congress of the World Association for Laser Therapy, Kansas City*: 34.

Schlager, A., T. Offer, and I. Baldissera. 1998. Laser stimulation of acupuncture point P6 reduces postoperative vomiting in children undergoing strabismus surgery. *British Journal of Anesthesia* 81, no. 4: 529-532.

Schoen, Allen M., ed. 1994. *Veterinary Acupuncture: Ancient Art to Modern Medicine*. St. Louis: Mosby, Inc.

Shamir, M. H., S. Rochkind, J. Sandbank, and M. Alon. 2001. Double-blind randomized study evaluating regeneration of the rat transected sciatic nerve after suturing and postoperative low-power laser treatment. *Journal of Reconstructive Microsurgery* 17, no. 2: 133-137.

Shiomi, Y., H. Takahashi, I. Honjo, H. Kojima, Y. Naito, and N. Fujiki. 1997. Efficacy of transmeatal low power laser irradition on tinnitus: A preliminary report. *Auris Nasus Larynx* 24, no. 1: 39-42.

Sidorov, V. D., D. R. Mamiliaeva, E. V. Gontar', S. Iu. Reformatskaia. 1999. [The interauricular laser therapy of rheumatoid arthritis.] *Voprosy Kurortologii, Fizioterapii, I Lechebnoi Fizicheskoi Kultury* 3: 35-43.

Simunovic, Z. 1996. Low level laser therapy with trigger points technique: A clinical study on 243 patients. *Journal of Clinical Laser Medicine and Surgery* 14, no. 4: 163-167.

Simunovic, Z., and T. Trobonjaca. 2000. Soft-tissue injuries from sport activities and traffic accidents – treatment with low-level laser therapy: A multicenter double-blind placebo-controlled clinical study on 132 patients. *Proceedings of SPIE* 4166: 286-293.

Simunovic, Z., A. D. Ivankovich, and A. Depolo. 2000. Wound healing of animal and human body sport and traffic accident injuries using low-level laser therapy treatment: A randomized clinical study of seventy-four patients with control group. *Journal of Clinical Laser Medicine and Surgery* 18, no. 2: 67-73.

Simunovic, Z., T. Trobonjaca, and Z. Trobonjaca. 1998. Treatment of medial and lateral epicondylitis – tennis and golfer's elbow – with low level laser therapy: A multicenter double-blind, placebo-controlled clinical study on 324 patients. *Journal of Clinical Laser Medicine and Surgery* 16, no. 3: 145-151.

70

Siposan, D., and A. Lukacs. 2000. Effect of low-level laser radiation on some rheological factors in human blood: An in vitro study. *Journal of Clinical Laser Medicine and Surgery* 18, no. 4: 185-195.

Siposan, D., and A. Lukacs. 2001. Relative variation to received dose of some erythrocytic and leukocytic indices of human blood as a result of low-level laser radiation: An in vitro study. *Journal of Clinical Laser Medicine and Surgery* 19, no. 2: 89-103.

Sroka, R., M. Schaffer, C. Fuchs, T. Pongratz, U. Schrader-Reichard, M. Busch, et al. 1999. Effects on the mitosis of normal and tumor cells induced by light treatment of different wavelengths. *Lasers in Surgery and Medicine* 25, no. 3: 263-271.

Stadler, I., R. Evans, B. Kolb, J. Naim, V. Narayan, N. Buehner, et al. 2000. In vitro effects of low-level laser irradiation at 660 nm on peripheral blood lymphocytes. *Lasers in Surgery and Medicine* 27, no. 3: 255-261.

Stadler, I., R. J. Lanzafame, R. Evans, V. Narayan, B. Dailey, N. Buehner, et al. 2001. 830-nm irradiation increases the wound tensile strength in a diabetic murine model. *Lasers in Surgery and Medicine* 28, no. 3: 220-226.

Stelian, J., I. Gil, B. Habot, M. Rosenthal, I. Abramovici, N. Kutok, et al. 1992. Improvement of pain and disability in elderly patients with degenerative osteoarthritis of the knee treated with narrow-band light therapy. *Journal of the American Geriatrics Society* 40: 23-26.

Taguchi, Y., and J. Maeda. 1998. Clinical experiences of laser applications in physical therapy. *Proceedings of the 2nd Congress of the World Association for Laser Therapy, Kansas City*: 106.

Tam, G. 1999. Low power laser therapy and analgesic action. *Journal of Clinical Laser Medicine and Surgery* 17, no.1: 29-33.

Tranquilli, William J., Kurt A. Grimm, and Leigh A. Lamont. 2000. *Pain Management for the Small Animal Practitioner*. Jackson, WY: Teton NewMedia.

Trojacanec, Z., S. Nikolic, and Z. Handziski. 1997. Low energy laser in the treatment of ulcus cruris. Abstract. *Abstracts of ICMART '97 International Medical Acupuncture Symposium*: 103.

Tsuchiya, K., M. Kawatani, C. Takeshige, T. Sato, and I. Matsumoto. 1993. Diode laser irradiation selectively diminishes slow component of axonal volley to dorsal roots from the saphenous nerve in the rat. *Neuroscience Letters* 161, no. 1: 65-68.

Tunér, J., and L. Hode. 1998. It's all in the parameters: A critical analysis of some well-known negative studies on low-level laser therapy. *Journal of Clinical Laser Medicine and Surgery* 16, no. 5: 245-248.

Tunér, J., and L. Hode. 2000. 100 double blind studies – enough or too little? *Proceedings of SPIE* 4166: 226-232.

Ueda, Y., and N. Shimizu. 2001. Pulse irradiation of low-power laser stimulates bone nodule formation. *Journal of Oral Science* 43, no. 1: 55-60.

Velizhanina, I. A., L. I. Gapon, M. S. Shabalina, and N. N. Kamalova. 2001. Efficiency of low-intensity laser radiation in essential hypertension. *Klinicheskaia Meditsina* 79, no. 1: 41-44.

Verdote-Robertson, R., M. M. Munchua, and J. R. Reddon. 2000. The use of low intensity laser therapy (LILT) for the treatment of open wounds in psychogeriatric patients: A pilot study. *Physical and Occupational Therapy in Geriatrics* 18, no. 2: 1-19.

Vin'kova, G. A., A.P. Ionin, and G. I. Ionina. 1999. [The treatment of posttraumatic uveitis with low-intensity laser radiation.] *Vestnik Oftalmologii* 115, no. 5: 20-21.

Webb, C., M. Dyson, and W. H. Lewis. 1998. Stimulatory effect of 660 nm low level laser energy on hypertrophic scar-derived fibroblasts: Possible mechanisms for increase in cell counts. *Lasers in Surgery and Medicine* 22, no. 5: 294-301.

Wilden, L., and R. Karthein. 1998. Import of radiation phenomena of electrons and therapeutic low-level laser in regard to the mitochondrial energy transfer. *Journal of Clinical Laser Medicine and Surgery* 16, no. 3: 159-165.

Wowapi Publishing. 2002. *Understanding Low Level Laser Therapy*. Portland, OR: Wowapi, Inc.

Wynn, Susan G., and Steve Marsden. 2003. *Manual of Natural Veterinary Medicine: Science and Tradition*. St. Louis: Mosby, Inc.

Xiaoa, X., J. Donga, X. Chua, J. Jiaob, S. Jiaa, X. Zhenga, et al. 2000-2001. A single photon emission computed tomography study of the therapy of intravascular low intensity laser irradiation on blood for brain infarction. Abstract. Millennium edition, *Journal of Laser Therapy* 13.

# INDEX

For more information, or if you would like to purchase a low-level laser or attend a low-level laser seminar, contact:

Dr. Tami Shearer
1306 Bethel Road
Columbus, Ohio 43220
614-457-2051
laservet@bright.net